THE HEALTHCARE CHAPLAIN'S JOURNEY

WITH AN END-OF-LIFE PATIENT

M. C. BROWN

COPYRIGHT©2025, M. C. BROWN

All rights reserved. No part of this publication may be reproduced, stored in a retrieval system, or transmitted in any form or by any means – electronic, mechanical, photocopy, recording, or any other except for brief quotations in printed reviews without permission of the publisher.

ISBN(PB): 979-8-89604-302-7

ISBN(HB): 978-1-9192226-2-2

Published by:

MANIFEST R819 PUBLICATIONS

UK: +44204538872

USA: +1(347)749-8363

Email: admin@manifestr819.com

www.manifestr819.com

CONTENTS

BOOK OVERVIEW 5
INTRODUCTION 13
   A CALLING BEYOND CURE 13
CHAPTER 1 17
   THE FIRST ENCOUNTER — MEETING THE PATIENT WHERE THEY ARE 17
CHAPTER 2 23
   BUILDING TRUST IN THE SHADOW OF DEATH 23
CHAPTER 3 29
   LISTENING DEEPLY — THE MINISTRY OF PRESENCE 29
CHAPTER 4 35
   SPIRITUAL PAIN AND UNFINISHED BUSINESS 35
CHAPTER 5 41
   WALKING WITH FAMILY — GRIEF BEFORE DEATH ... 41
CHAPTER 6 47
   FAITH CONVERSATIONS AT THE THRESHOLD 47
CHAPTER 7 53
   ETHICAL CHALLENGES AND INTERDISCIPLINARY TENSIONS 53
CHAPTER 8 59
   THE SACREDNESS OF SILENCE AND RITUALS 59

CHAPTER 9 65
  THE FINAL HOURS — HOLDING SPACE FOR DEPARTURE 65

CHAPTER 10 71
  AFTER DEATH — BLESSING, COMMITTAL, AND CONTINUING CARE 71

CHAPTER 11 79
  THE CHAPLAIN'S OWN GRIEF AND GROWTH 79

CHAPTER 12 85
  REFLECTIONS ON PRACTICE — THEOLOGICAL AND PRACTICAL INSIGHTS 85

CONCLUSION 93
  DEATH AS HOLY GROUND 93

APPENDICES 97
  APPENDIX A: SAMPLE PRAYERS AND BLESSINGS 97

BOOK OVERVIEW

Introduction — A Calling Beyond Cure

Healthcare chaplaincy at the end of life is not a ministry of miracles but of presence. While medicine aims to extend life, chaplaincy honours the mystery of its ending. The chaplain is not there to fix, but to witness, to hold, and to accompany. This book is a narrative, theological, and pastoral reflection on that sacred journey, of one chaplain with one dying patient, and what that story teaches us about dignity, faith, and what it means to truly accompany someone into the arms of eternity.

CHAPTER 1: THE FIRST ENCOUNTER — MEETING THE PATIENT WHERE THEY ARE

Every end-of-life journey begins with a meeting, tentative, uncertain. The patient, let's call him Kojo, had been diagnosed with terminal cancer. He was angry, not at God, but at what he called "the silence of it all." The first visit was short. No prayer. Just presence. A chair pulled close; silence shared. This is where the journey began, with listening, not speaking.

CHAPTER 2: BUILDING TRUST IN THE SHADOW OF DEATH

Over time, Kojo began to open up. "I don't need someone to convert me," he said. "I need someone to hear me." And that was my role: to build trust, slowly, respectfully. Trust was not a tool but a grace. It allowed for sacred conversations about guilt, regret, love, and hope.

CHAPTER 3: LISTENING DEEPLY — THE MINISTRY OF PRESENCE

The heart of chaplaincy is not talking, but listening. Deep, empathetic, non-anxious listening. Kojo shared stories of his estranged daughter. Of a faith he once knew. Of songs he missed singing. Each word was sacred. The room became holy ground.

CHAPTER 4: SPIRITUAL PAIN AND UNFINISHED BUSINESS

"I feel like I left things undone," Kojo said. Spiritual pain is real, a sense of disconnection from God, others, or self. Together, we explored forgiveness. Not as a forced ritual, but as a courageous step. One day, he asked for a phone to call his daughter. That call was not magic. But it was holy.

CHAPTER 5: WALKING WITH FAMILY — GRIEF BEFORE DEATH

His daughter came. Their reunion was quiet, tearful. As chaplain, I supported not only Kojo but his family. Anticipatory grief is real, mourning begins before death. Through family conversations, shared readings, and even just tea and silence, chaplaincy created a space for grace.

CHAPTER 6: FAITH CONVERSATIONS AT THE THRESHOLD

Kojo began to ask about God again. "Is He still listening?" he asked. We read Psalm 23. He remembered the lines from childhood. We didn't argue theology. We prayed. He asked for anointing. The oil wasn't a miracle cure. But in that moment, it was everything.

CHAPTER 7: ETHICAL CHALLENGES AND INTERDISCIPLINARY TENSIONS

Not everyone on the care team understood spiritual care. "What does the chaplain actually do?" some asked. There were tensions around assisted dying conversations, spiritual assessments, and family requests. The chaplain's role is to advocate for dignity, meaning, and the patient's voice, especially when medicine can go no further.

CHAPTER 8: THE SACREDNESS OF SILENCE AND RITUALS

Sometimes there were no words. Just hand-holding, humming, silent prayers. Rituals, reading a Psalm, lighting a candle, offering a blessing, grounded us. Ritual isn't just religious; it's relational. It reminds us that death is not just clinical, it's sacred.

CHAPTER 9: THE FINAL HOURS — HOLDING SPACE FOR DEPARTURE

The room was dim. Family gathered. Kojo asked for Psalm 121. I read. He closed his eyes. His breathing slowed. We sang softly. Then silence. In those final moments, chaplaincy was about holding space, not fixing, not preaching, just being there. He passed away in peace.

CHAPTER 10: AFTER DEATH — BLESSING, COMMITTAL, AND CONTINUING CARE

After death, chaplaincy continues. With words, with presence, with ritual. I blessed the body. I comforted the family. I helped staff process. End-of-life care does not end at death. The chaplain is there to honour both departure and the living left behind.

CHAPTER 11: THE CHAPLAIN'S OWN GRIEF AND GROWTH

Chaplaincy touches the chaplain. I wept for Kojo. Not as a therapist, but as a companion. We do not leave untouched. But in grief, there is growth, a deeper compassion, a renewed calling. Each patient leaves a mark, a silent teaching.

CHAPTER 12: REFLECTIONS ON PRACTICE — THEOLOGICAL AND PRACTICAL INSIGHTS

This work draws on Christian theology, interfaith respect, palliative principles, and pastoral care skills. Scripture like Romans 8, Revelation 21, and John 14 inform our hope. But so too do dignity, ethics, and humanity. The chaplain walks between worlds, between hospital and heaven.

CONCLUSION — DEATH AS HOLY GROUND

Chaplaincy at the end of life is sacred work. It is where theology meets touch, where doctrine meets dying. It is not about eloquence, but presence. Not about having answers, but about honouring questions. In the dying moment, the chaplain is not a preacher but a companion. And in that companionship, the divine draws near.

APPENDICES

A. Sample Prayers and Blessings
- Prayers for Peace
- Prayer for the Dying
- Interfaith Final Blessing

B. Interfaith Considerations
- Ministering with respect to different beliefs
- Collaborating with faith leaders
- Cultural sensitivity at end-of-life

C. Chaplain Self-Care
- Debriefing with peers
- Reflective journaling
- Spiritual direction

INTRODUCTION

A CALLING BEYOND CURE

There are moments in healthcare when medicine meets its limits. No surgery can be performed. No treatment will change the outcome. No prescription will restore life. It is in these moments, raw, sacred, and final, that the ministry of the healthcare chaplain begins. This is the threshold between life and death, where physical care gives way to spiritual presence.

Chaplaincy is not about fixing. It is not about controlling outcomes, prescribing faith, or offering platitudes. It is about being there. It is a ministry of presence, simple, often silent, always sacred. The chaplain enters into the most vulnerable of human experiences: pain, dying, grief, regret, love, and hope. We walk beside, never in front. We accompany, not command. We listen, not lecture.

The end-of-life journey is one of complexity and depth. For the patient, it may be a time of reflection, fear, anticipation, or even peace. For the family, it often includes grief before death, anticipatory mourning for what is already being lost. For the medical team, it is a moment to honour life, even as it slips away. And for the chaplain, it is a sacred calling, a pastoral privilege that touches the eternal.

This book is a reflection on that journey. It tells the story of one chaplain and one patient. Yet, in that story are countless others: every man or woman who has faced the end; every soul who has asked, *"Am I alone?"*; and every spiritual caregiver who has sat at the bedside, holding space for a mystery beyond words.

My purpose in writing is both personal and professional. As a chaplain, I have been transformed by walking with those at the end of life. As a minister of faith, I have witnessed how the divine often draws near in dying moments, sometimes in prayer, sometimes in silence. As a human being, I have come to see death not as failure, but as a transition, a holy passage that invites reverence, not fear.

Too often, the spiritual dimensions of dying are neglected or treated as secondary. Hospitals may be full of machines and monitors, but what of meaning? What of hope? What of the unseen wounds, guilt, shame, unfinished business, spiritual distress? These are not questions for physicians alone. They are questions for the soul, and for those who care for the soul.

In the chapters that follow, you will journey with me through real experiences and reflections from the bedside of a terminally ill patient. You will encounter spiritual struggles, ethical dilemmas, moments of reconciliation, and the quiet presence of the sacred. The language will be pastoral, the theology accessible, and the tone honest, for there is no pretending in the face of death.

This is not a manual, though it offers insight. It is not a memoir, though it is deeply personal. It is a pastoral-theological exploration of what it means to walk with another towards the end of life, and what that journey teaches us about living, dying, and the God who meets us in both.

Above all, this book is a tribute, to the patient who allowed me to walk with him; to the countless others I have had the privilege of serving; and to the sacred work of healthcare chaplaincy.

Welcome to the journey.

CHAPTER 1

THE FIRST ENCOUNTER — MEETING THE PATIENT WHERE THEY ARE

Every journey has a beginning. In healthcare chaplaincy, that beginning is rarely scheduled, polished, or predictable. It often comes unannounced, in the midst of the ordinary routines of a hospital, and in moments that feel raw and unprepared. The first meeting with an end-of-life patient is not a rehearsed exchange or a carefully staged event; it is an entrance into sacred space, into someone else's pain, questions, and reality. It demands not only professional skill, but also sensitivity, humility, and spiritual discernment.

I still remember the first time I met Kojo. His name had been passed to me quietly by the palliative care nurse. She leaned in slightly and spoke in a low voice:

"He's been given a few weeks. You might try him. He hasn't asked for a chaplain, but he might benefit from a visit."

In healthcare settings, that phrase, *might benefit*, often carries more weight than it seems. It is sometimes code for: *He's struggling in ways we cannot quite name, and we hope you might help.*

I made my way to his room, knocked gently, and stepped inside. Kojo was lying on his side, facing away from the door. The television was on but muted, its flickering light playing across the walls. The air felt heavy, not just with the presence of illness, but with something deeper: an emotional density, a kind of spiritual weight that is hard to name yet immediately felt.

I introduced myself softly.

"Kojo, I'm Michael, the chaplain here. I just came to say hello. I won't stay long."

There was no verbal welcome. Just a faint grunt. But importantly, he did not ask me to leave.

I found a chair and sat, not too close, not too far. I stayed still. Said nothing. Sometimes, the most important ministry in a first encounter is not found in words, but in silence. Silence, when held with respect, has a language of its own. It speaks without intrusion. It allows the patient to set the pace.

Several minutes passed before he turned his head slightly, catching sight of me for the first time.

"So, you're the God guy?" he asked.

I smiled gently.

"I'm here for spiritual support. For whatever you need."

He gave a dry chuckle.

"What I need is to not be dying."

I nodded, meeting his gaze without flinching.

"That makes a lot of sense."

He seemed almost taken aback that I didn't rush in with explanations, Bible verses, or hollow assurances. I didn't try to fix his statement or soften it. I simply acknowledged it for what it was, a truth from his perspective, voiced with honesty.

That moment shifted something. He wasn't ready for prayer. He wasn't sure what he believed anymore. But he also didn't ask me to go. That was enough for now.

The first encounter in chaplaincy is about permission, not performance. It is about offering the patient a measure of control in a world where so much has already been taken from them. They did not choose their illness. They did not plan to die so soon. They did not request the chaplain's presence. Therefore, any offering of spiritual care must begin with consent, given gently, patiently, and respectfully.

In that first meeting, chaplains listen with more than ears. We listen with our posture, with the tone of our voice, with the silences we allow. We listen by noticing the room: the family photographs on the shelf, the wilting flowers in a vase, the well-worn Bible or perhaps the absence of anything spiritual at all. We enter as guests into sacred space, space that belongs entirely to the patient, and we tread with care.

Kojo did not want to talk long. After about ten minutes, he said,

"You can go now."

It was not said with hostility, only with honesty. I stood, thanked him, and assured him that I would check in again.

That was all.

But that brief visit became the foundation for everything that followed. In its own quiet way, it communicated respect, presence, and availability. It said: *You are not alone. When you are ready, I will be here.*

In chaplaincy, the first encounter is never about solving problems or delivering profound truths. It is about showing up, not as the answer, but as a companion. And sometimes, that simple act of presence is the true beginning of everything that matters.

CHAPTER 2

BUILDING TRUST IN THE SHADOW OF DEATH

Trust is not freely handed to strangers; it is earned. And in the hospital room of a dying patient, that truth is magnified. Especially when that patient did not request your presence. Especially when faith, once vibrant, has become tangled with disappointment, loss, or unanswered questions. As chaplains, we do not step into such spaces as spiritual engineers with ready-made blueprints. We arrive as fellow travellers, strangers at first, and if we are wise, humble ones.

My second visit with Kojo felt different from the first. Still reserved, but no longer closed, he looked up as I entered. This time, there was no trace of surprise in his eyes.

"You again," he said, before adding with a faint nod, "You didn't push too hard last time. I appreciated that."

It was only a small acknowledgement, but to me it was significant, the first step across the fragile bridge of trust.

We spoke for perhaps twenty minutes. He told me about his years as a schoolteacher, thirty in total. He loved history. Loved working with children. His voice carried a quiet pride when speaking of his career. Then, as if sliding over a shadow, he mentioned that he had never remarried after his divorce. He had one daughter.

"We don't talk much," he said, the words landing flat.

I didn't push. I simply nodded, letting the moment be.

Almost as an afterthought, he added,

"I used to go to church. But after my brother died… I don't know. I just kind of stopped."

He looked away towards the window, his gaze fixed somewhere beyond the glass.

"I don't think God cared much."

I didn't rush in to defend God or offer theological explanations. I simply asked,

"Did you tell Him that?"

His head turned back towards me, a half-smile touching his lips.

"No. I just stopped talking altogether."

This is where trust is born, in the quiet, unhurried moments where people discover they can speak without fear of being corrected, preached at, or smothered in optimism. Too often, those approaching the end of life find themselves surrounded by people eager to *fix* them, inspire them, or save them. But Kojo wasn't asking to be saved. He wanted someone who could be with him without conditions, who could hold the truth of his pain without flinching.

Over the weeks that followed, he began to share more. He spoke of his regrets and his hopes. He told me about the music he loved, his distant relationship with his daughter, and his dislike of being pitied.

"I'm dying," he said once, "but I'm still a person. Not a project."

That line lodged itself in my mind: *Not a project.* It is a reminder every chaplain needs to hear. We must resist the temptation to see patients as cases to be managed or assignments to be completed. They are whole people, with complexity, depth, and their own rhythm of trust.

Building that trust took consistency. I visited regularly, even when he didn't have much to say. I asked before offering prayer. I honoured his boundaries. I made sure that if I said I would come, I came. Slowly, the guarded edges softened.

One afternoon, he looked at me and said,

"You know, I look forward to your visits. Not because you talk about God. But because you don't try to sell Him to me."

It was, perhaps, the highest praise I could receive from a man who had once turned his back on faith.

Trust is not built on eloquence. It is built on authenticity. It grows through presence, patience, and integrity. In the shadow of death, trust becomes the bridge across which sacred conversations can walk, sometimes hesitantly, sometimes boldly, but always more freely than before.

Chaplains are not magicians. We do not mend the reality of dying. But we can offer something that medicine, for all its skill, cannot, a trustworthy presence in a world that has become uncertain. And often, it is that steady presence that opens the heart to hope, to healing of the unseen kind, and to the peace that quietly waits at the end of the journey.

CHAPTER 3

LISTENING DEEPLY — THE MINISTRY OF PRESENCE

If there is one core practice that defines the chaplain's role at the end of life, it is this: listening. Not passive hearing. Not politely waiting for a pause to insert our own words. But deep, attentive, empathic listening, the kind that welcomes a person to be fully seen, fully heard, and fully honoured, even in their dying.

With Kojo, our visits gradually grew more open. His words began to reach beyond his medical condition and into the territory of the soul. He spoke of the silence of the hospital room at night, how it seemed to settle on him like a blanket, heavy and unshakable.

He described the strange way time seemed to stretch, each minute dragging as if reluctant to move. He shared his dreams, both the ones that visited him in the quiet hours of sleep and the ones that belonged to his past and future. And slowly, he began to name fears that had previously remained locked away.

What Kojo needed from me was not advice. It was not tidy answers to theological mysteries. It was something far more demanding: the willingness to hold his words exactly as they were, without trying to reshape or fix them.

One afternoon, he said quietly:

"I dreamed about my brother again. He was sitting by a river, humming an old hymn. I could see his face, peaceful, like he used to be. Then I woke up and couldn't stop crying. Do you think that means something?"

I resisted the temptation to interpret or spiritualise. Instead, I replied,

"It sounds like that moment meant something to you. Would you like to talk more about him?"

And he did.

Deep listening is a form of spiritual hospitality. It opens the door of the soul and says, *You are safe here. Speak what you need to speak. You will not be judged, hurried, or shut down.* It is one of the greatest gifts we can offer someone approaching death, especially when so much else in their life is already being taken from them.

There were times when Kojo's voice would falter mid-sentence, emotions swelling and spilling over. Sometimes he wept. Sometimes he laughed at a half-forgotten memory. And sometimes, he said nothing at all, staring out of the window as though looking for something beyond the horizon. I learnt to welcome those silences instead of fearing them.

In chaplaincy, silence is not emptiness. It is space, space in which the soul can breathe. The dying do not always need to be filled with words; they need to know they are not alone in the quiet.

One day, after an especially raw conversation about his daughter and the regrets he carried, Kojo looked at me and said,

"You don't look away. Most people do. But you sit with it. Why?"

I paused before answering.

"Because this is sacred. And sacred things are worth honouring."

That simple exchange reminded me: presence itself is ministry. The ability to remain with someone in their grief, not rushing to fix, not recoiling from their pain, is one of the rarest and most powerful expressions of love.

In healthcare systems that so often hurry, measure, and prescribe, the chaplain's role is quietly countercultural. We are called to slow down. To stay. To see the person when others are focused only on the patient. To listen for the soul while others attend to the body.

Listening deeply creates space for meaning to emerge. It allows for memories to be cherished, for truth to be spoken, for reconciliation to take place, sometimes with others, sometimes with oneself, and sometimes with God.

In Kojo's case, it gave him a language for his inner world. He told me once,

"I didn't know I needed to say these things, until someone gave me the space to say them."

And that is the ministry of presence. It is not loud, not dramatic, and never flashy. It is steady, faithful, and profoundly human. It is the art of being with someone as they find their own words, their own peace, and perhaps even their own healing, all in the quiet company of one who will not turn away.

CHAPTER 4

SPIRITUAL PAIN AND UNFINISHED BUSINESS

Not all suffering is physical. In the stillness of end-of-life care, another kind of pain often emerges, harder to name, harder to treat, but just as real. It is *spiritual pain*.

Spiritual pain comes in many forms: guilt over past actions or inactions; deep regret for words left unsaid or relationships left broken; a loss of meaning or purpose; fear of the unknown; a sense of disconnection from God, from others, or even from oneself. Sometimes it takes the form of a haunting question, *Has my life truly mattered?* or a gnawing feeling that something essential remains unresolved. For many, this inner anguish can weigh more heavily than the physical illness itself.

Kojo began to speak more openly about these deeper wounds.

"I feel like I left things undone," he admitted one afternoon. "Like I missed something important, but it's too late to fix it now."

He lay back on the pillow, staring at the ceiling, his hands folded across his chest, a posture that seemed equal parts resignation and protection.

I asked softly,

"What do you feel was left undone?"

There was a pause, as if the words were fragile and needed careful handling. Then came the slow, halting confession.

"My daughter. We haven't spoken in years. I let the divorce come between us. I didn't fight for her. And now I'm here, dying… and she's out there, and I don't know if she even cares."

I allowed the silence to settle between us. Pain had risen to the surface, and silence gave it room to breathe. Beneath that pain, I sensed a possibility, the first small opening towards healing.

Spiritual pain often reveals what is most sacred to the person. For Kojo, it was not doctrinal questions or theological arguments that surfaced. It was relationship. A broken bond. A longing for connection. And under the weight of sorrow, there was still a flicker of hope, the faint belief that perhaps it was not too late.

We spoke about forgiveness, not as an abstract theological term, but as a lived, difficult, deeply human process.

"It's not just about being forgiven," I told him gently. "Sometimes, it's also about forgiving yourself."

He shook his head slowly.

"Easier said than done."

"Yes," I agreed, "but maybe you don't have to do it alone."

Over the next few visits, the subject of his daughter returned again and again, like a tide that could not be held back. At first, he circled it cautiously, unwilling to risk the pain of hope. But something was changing. His words began to lose their bitterness, replaced instead by sorrow, and sorrow, in turn, made space for grace.

Then, one day, without prompting, he asked quietly,

"Do you think…do you think you could help me write something to her?"

I felt the significance of the moment.

"Of course," I said. "Whenever you're ready."

That letter became a turning point. He dictated; I wrote. It was not a polished apology. It was not an attempt to explain away the years. But it was heartfelt, an honest reaching across the gap. When we sealed the envelope and posted it together, it felt as though we had placed something sacred into the hands of God.

Two days later, she called the hospital. And the next morning, she arrived.

Their reunion was tentative at first, quiet, almost awkward. Then the barriers gave way. They held hands. They cried. They forgave. And they said what needed to be said.

Was everything neatly resolved? No. Life rarely grants us tidy endings. But something holy had happened: the spiritual wound had been named, honoured, and partially healed.

This is the essence of chaplaincy, not to fix people or force closure, but to walk alongside them as they do the courageous work of reconciling with themselves, with others, and, sometimes, with God.

Spiritual pain is holy ground. It cannot be rushed through with quick prayers or dismissed with platitudes. It must be entered with reverence, explored with gentleness, and accompanied with hope wherever possible.

Kojo still carried some sorrow. But now, he was no longer carrying it alone. And sometimes, that is the difference between despair and peace.

CHAPTER 5

WALKING WITH FAMILY — GRIEF BEFORE DEATH

When someone is dying, the weight of suffering does not rest on them alone. Those who love them walk their own road of pain, a path often unseen and unspoken, but no less real. As chaplains, our calling extends not only to the patient, but also to those who wait at the bedside, those who grieve in advance, and those who will carry the loss into the days beyond.

Kojo's daughter, Ama, came to the hospital hesitantly. Their relationship had been fractured for more than a decade. The letter he had dictated and sent broke the long silence between them, but the years of distance still hung in the air. She entered the room quietly, clutching a small bag in one hand and the weight of disappointment in the other.

I stepped out to give them space. When I returned some time later, they were sitting together in subdued conversation. The air felt different. Tears had been shed, words had been spoken, and something fragile yet unmistakably real had begun, a reconnection not built on perfect resolution, but on grace.

Over the following days, Ama became a regular presence in the room. She brought photographs, small tokens of shared history. She asked gentle questions. She laughed softly at some memories, and at other times, I found her in the hallway with tears running down her face.

Once, while Kojo slept, she turned to me and said quietly, "I wasn't ready for this. I thought we had more time."

Grief begins long before death. This anticipatory grief, the sorrow of impending loss, can be as intense and disorienting as the grief that follows after a loved one's passing. It may arrive as sadness, anger, anxiety, exhaustion, or guilt. For many families, the hospital becomes a place of paradox: a sanctuary of care, and at the same time, a place of slow heartbreak.

Part of my ministry was to walk with Ama in her grief as well. Not just as Kojo's daughter, but as a woman navigating her own "valley of the shadow".

We spoke often. Sometimes for five minutes, sometimes for longer stretches. I listened as she untangled years of silence, recent moments of forgiveness, and the raw ache of watching her father weaken. I did not try to explain away her feelings or rush her to acceptance. I simply held space for her to feel what she needed to feel.

Other family members began to appear, a niece, an old friend from Kojo's teaching days. Each brought their own memories, their own unresolved emotions. The chaplain's role in these moments is to be a safe harbour in that sea of uncertainty, a presence outside the family's history, but fully within its most vulnerable season.

One morning, sensing Ama's weariness, I brought a small printed prayer card and asked, "Would you like me to read this blessing with you?"

She nodded.

The words were simple, not overtly religious, but deeply human and comforting. As I read, tears rolled freely down her cheeks. When I finished, she whispered,

"That's what I needed. Just that."

Spiritual care for families is not about taking sides, giving advice, or solving the unsolvable. It is about presence, permission, and peace. It is about helping them discover their own way of showing love, of saying goodbye, and of making meaning in the midst of loss.

As Kojo's condition declined, Ama's care for him became almost instinctive. She adjusted his pillows. She held his hand during restless spells. She whispered prayers when his own voice failed him. In these moments, their relationship, though different from what either might once have imagined, became something redemptive, tender, and true.

When families are supported during the dying process, their grief after death often feels more anchored. They can say, with quiet assurance: *I was there. I loved. I said what mattered.*

The chaplain in these moments does not stand apart, observing from the margins. We stand alongside. We bring tissues, offer chairs, fetch water, suggest a prayer, hold the silence, and, above all, embody presence with compassion.

To walk with a patient is holy work. To walk with their family is holy, too.

CHAPTER 6

FAITH CONVERSATIONS AT THE THRESHOLD

As the end of life approaches, questions of faith often rise to the surface. They rarely come neatly packaged in theological language; more often, they are raw, human expressions of longing, fear, or fragile hope. Some patients return to a faith they once abandoned. Others wrestle with doubts that have never been voiced aloud. Many wonder, silently or openly: *Is God here? Does He still care? What happens when I die?*

Kojo had been ambivalent about faith throughout much of our time together. Raised in the church, he had walked away decades earlier after the sudden death of his brother.

"I just couldn't believe in a God who let that happen," he told me once, his voice still heavy with the memory.

But as his body weakened and the horizon of life grew near, his resistance began to soften. The questions returned, not in defiance, but in a quiet, searching way.

One afternoon, he sat gazing out of the hospital window at a sky thick with grey clouds. Without turning to me, he asked,

"Do you think He still hears me, after all these years of silence?"

It was not a rhetorical question. It was a plea from somewhere deep within.

"I believe He never stopped listening," I said softly. "Even in the silence. Even in the anger."

He nodded slowly, letting the words rest in the air between us.

These moments are not about persuasion or theological debate. They are sacred thresholds, places where the chaplain is called to tread lightly, reverently, and truthfully. Faith at the edge of life is seldom built on argument; it is nurtured through presence, trust, and gentle invitation.

Over the next few visits, Kojo asked if we could read Scripture together.

"I don't remember much," he confessed with a faint smile. "Just a few lines from the Psalms... something about a shepherd?"

"Psalm 23," I replied. "Would you like to hear it?"

He nodded.

As I began, *"The Lord is my shepherd, I shall not want...",* he closed his eyes. When I reached the words, *"Even though I walk through the valley of the shadow of death, I will fear no evil,"* a tear slid slowly down his cheek.

"Can we read that again?" he whispered.

We did. And when the words came a second time, they seemed to settle over him like a warm covering.

Faith conversations at the end of life are rarely structured or formal. They are tender, deeply personal, and often shaped by the smallest of moments: a remembered hymn, a whispered prayer, a question long avoided but now given voice. They may involve Scripture, prayer, confession, or the sacraments, but more often they happen quietly, woven into ordinary conversation.

One evening, Kojo asked, "Would it be okay if you anointed me? Like in the old days?"

I smiled, moved by the request.

"Of course," I said. "It would be my honour."

The next day, I brought a small vial of oil. I explained the meaning of the anointing, a blessing, a sign of God's presence, a prayer for peace. Then I traced the sign of the cross on his forehead and hands, praying softly. The prayer was not for healing in the physical sense, but for peace, courage, and surrender.

The atmosphere in the room shifted. It felt as though the space itself had become sacred ground. Kojo looked at me afterwards and said,

"I feel lighter. Not fixed, but seen."

That is what faith can offer in dying moments: not every answer, not the removal of every fear, but a deep sense of being held, noticed, and not alone.

As chaplains, our task is never to force faith or impose belief. It is to honour what is present, whether a long-held conviction, a tentative question, or a deeply felt absence. We meet people where they are: Christian, Muslim, Jewish, Hindu, agnostic, atheist, or uncertain. And we create space for the sacred to surface in whatever way it wishes.

Faith, at the threshold of death, is less about doctrine and more about relationship, with God, with oneself, with one's past, and with those who remain. It is about naming what matters. About remembering that life had meaning. About daring to trust, however faintly, that something holy waits on the other side.

For Kojo, faith returned not as a sudden blaze, but as a small flame, flickering, yet real. And in his final days, that flame offered warmth, comfort, and the courage to face the unknown.

CHAPTER 7

ETHICAL CHALLENGES AND INTERDISCIPLINARY TENSIONS

The role of the chaplain in healthcare is both spiritual and relational, but it is also institutional. We move within complex systems, shaped by clinical protocols, legal frameworks, professional boundaries, and unspoken cultural norms. While chaplains are often welcomed as sources of emotional and spiritual support, our presence can also stir deeper, sometimes uncomfortable, questions about how we care, why we care, and what truly matters when a life is nearing its end.

In Kojo's case, one of the first tensions emerged during a routine interdisciplinary meeting. The medical team reviewed his worsening prognosis. One nurse asked quietly,

"Should we offer him the option of palliative sedation?"

Another replied, "He hasn't asked. And I'm not sure how much he understands."

I listened for a while, weighing my words. Then, when the conversation paused, I spoke gently: "He's been expressing spiritual distress as well, regrets, unresolved family matters. He might need more than medication right now. He might need meaning."

Some heads nodded in agreement; others remained neutral. A few faces betrayed uncertainty about my place in the discussion. It is a familiar tension. Chaplains are not clinicians, but we are part of the team. We cannot prescribe treatment, yet we help assess the patient's spiritual readiness, emotional state, and existential pain. These are not side issues; they often shape how a patient receives care, how they make decisions, and how they face the reality of dying.

A particularly delicate ethical moment came later, when a member of Kojo's extended family spoke to me privately: "He doesn't want to be resuscitated, but what if we do? Can we override that?"

I replied, firmly but with compassion, "No. If he is of sound mind and has made that decision, it must be respected, by family and by staff."

They did not find the answer easy to hear. But part of ethical chaplaincy is advocacy, being a voice for the patient when their voice is at risk of being diminished. Advocacy is not about taking sides; it is about safeguarding dignity.

There were challenges from other directions, too. A staff member once asked, "Why is he spending so much time with the chaplain? He hasn't gone to church in years."

This is a subtle but persistent assumption: that spiritual care is only for the devout. The truth is, faith is not a prerequisite for soul care. Every human being, regardless of belief or religious identity, carries questions, values, longings, and stories. Chaplaincy is not about enforcing a creed; it is about recognising and honouring the human spirit in moments of vulnerability.

Kojo himself once voiced similar uncertainty: "I feel like I'm not religious enough for this. Like I missed my chance."

I looked at him and said, "You're here. And that's enough. God meets us where we are, not where we think we should have been."

Another sensitive area we sometimes encounter is assisted dying. While it was not legal in our context, patients occasionally raised it, especially when pain, fatigue, and hopelessness converged. Kojo never asked directly, but one day he sighed and said, "If I were a dog, they'd put me down by now. Why does death have to be so drawn out for humans?"

I did not debate. I did not preach. I acknowledged the depth of his weariness and stayed with him in it. Sometimes, the most ethical response is not a moral argument, but a compassionate presence that affirms: *I hear you. I see you. I am with you.*

Chaplains inhabit the space between disciplines, medicine, ethics, theology, psychology. We do not claim to have all the answers, but we must remain anchored: grounded in our calling, in our values, and in the courage to speak when the soul's needs risk being overlooked.

In healthcare, tensions are inevitable: between cure and comfort, between doing and being, between professional detachment and authentic compassion. The chaplain stands at that intersection, bearing witness to both the science and the sacred, not as an outsider, but as one who belongs to both worlds.

Kojo never needed me to resolve the system. He needed me to be present within it, for him. And that, in the end, was enough.

CHAPTER 8

THE SACREDNESS OF SILENCE AND RITUALS

There are moments in the chaplain's journey when words fail. Not because there is nothing to say, but because no words are sufficient. In such moments, silence ceases to be awkward and becomes sacred. And rituals, simple, meaningful acts, speak with a depth and clarity that language cannot match.

As Kojo's condition declined, our conversations grew shorter. Sometimes he was too tired to speak; other times, we simply sat together in quiet. Yet it was never an empty quiet. It was a silence filled with trust, with presence, with the deep assurance that someone was there, even if no words were exchanged.

Silence, when honoured, becomes a spiritual practice. It allows space for the soul to surface, unhurried and unforced. It creates room for unspoken grief, gentle reflection, or a peaceful surrender.

One afternoon, as the machines kept their steady rhythm and sunlight filtered softly through the blinds, Kojo opened his eyes and said, "Can we just sit today? No talking. Just be here."

"Of course," I replied.

And so we sat. Five minutes passed. Then ten. Then more. The world seemed to slow. The air felt still. And in that holy silence, Kojo drifted into sleep, peaceful, unafraid, and not alone.

As words began to fade, rituals came to the fore. Rituals are not mere traditions; they are embodied prayers, tangible acts that give shape to the spiritual, that make visible the invisible, that honour the holy without demanding explanation.

Kojo loved music, so one day I asked if he would like to hear a favourite hymn.

"Amazing Grace," he whispered.

I played it softly on my phone. He closed his eyes. A tear slid down his cheek, not from sadness, but from recognising something beautiful, familiar, and eternal.

Other small rituals followed. With the ward's permission, I lit a candle at his bedside. I read aloud from the Psalms. When his hands grew too weak to move, I traced the sign of the cross upon them for him.

These rituals grounded us. They reminded both Kojo and me that something sacred was taking place, that this was not merely the closing of a biological process, but a spiritual transition: a passing from one realm to another.

Rituals also became a gift to his family. One afternoon, his daughter Ama asked quietly,

"Can we do something together before he goes?"

I suggested a blessing. We gathered around his bed, held hands, and spoke words of peace, gratitude, and release. Tears fell freely. Yet, alongside the tears, there was a sense of completion, a gentle letting go.

Over the years, I have learned that people rarely remember the exact words a chaplain speaks. What they remember is how you were with them, the stillness you offered, the kindness you embodied, the hand you held, the hymn you played, the silence you shared.

And rituals do not need to be explicitly religious to be sacred. A moment of hand-holding. A shared reading. A whispered *"thank you"* or *"I love you."* These are not merely gestures; they are acts of honour, tokens of love, and signs of transcendence.

As Kojo's final days approached, the rituals became fewer, simpler, and more profound. A hand on his shoulder. A brief prayer. A presence that did not waver. Above all, a reverent silence that said without saying: *This moment matters. You matter. You are not alone.*

In the sacredness of silence and the simplicity of ritual, the chaplain becomes less a speaker and more a steward, of presence, of peace, and of holy ground.

CHAPTER 9

THE FINAL HOURS — HOLDING SPACE FOR DEPARTURE

There comes a moment in every end-of-life journey when time itself seems to hold its breath, when the air grows still, voices become hushed, and the sacred weight of the inevitable settles over the room like a gentle veil. These are the final hours.

Nothing can prepare you for them entirely. No training, no textbook, no prior experience can capture their depth. And yet, as chaplains, we are called to be fully present within this holy space. Not to control. Not to fix. But simply to hold space, to stand as a quiet witness to a mystery that is both deeply human and profoundly divine.

Kojo's final hours came gently, without struggle or haste. In the last two days of his life, his body began to withdraw from the world. He slept more, spoke less. His hands grew cool. His voice, when he used it, was little more than a whisper. His daughter, Ama, remained by his side almost constantly, her presence a soft anchor in the ebbing tide of time. I stayed too.

The room itself seemed to change. It became a sanctuary, quiet, dim, and tender, filled with murmured reassurances and occasional prayers. The soft hum of the medical equipment faded into the background, no longer the focus. Technology was still present, but its importance had diminished. We had entered a new rhythm, not of medicine, but of mystery.

Ama turned to me at one point, her eyes wide with both fear and love.

"Is this… is this it?"

I nodded gently. "Yes. He's close now. We'll just be with him."

Being with someone in their final hours is a ministry distilled to its purest essence. It is about presence without pressure. It is about staying calm when others feel unsettled. It is offering tissues, adjusting a chair, holding a hand, murmuring a word of comfort, or simply remaining silent, letting your presence speak what words cannot.

At one point, Kojo stirred. His eyes opened briefly, scanning the room until they rested on Ama. Then on me. With visible effort, he whispered, "Psalm…"

I knew. I reached for my Bible and read from Psalm 121: *"I lift up my eyes to the mountains, where does my help come from? My help comes from the Lord, the Maker of heaven and earth…"*

Kojo's eyes closed again, and his breathing slowed. A single tear traced its way down his cheek.

In the remaining hours, we surrounded him with the sounds and words he loved. Hymns played softly, each note a thread of comfort. Short prayers were spoken, prayers of peace, of gratitude, of release. We told him he was loved. That he was not alone. That it was all right to rest.

There is a rhythm to dying that the body knows. Breaths grow shallower, then irregular. Long pauses appear between them. Eyes may open briefly, as if seeing something beyond the room, before closing again. Then comes the stillness, the pause that does not end.

When Kojo took his final breath, the moment was unmistakable.

Ama bent forward, resting her forehead against his hand, tears soaking her cheeks. Her sobs were quiet, almost reverent. I placed my hand gently on his head and prayed aloud: "Into Your hands, O Lord, we commend Your servant. Receive him into Your eternal peace. May light perpetual shine upon him."

We did not rush. There was no need. Time was allowed to stand still for a little longer. Ama held her father's hand. I stayed close. Eventually, we informed the nursing staff. Together, we honoured his body with a final blessing. not out of routine alone, but out of deep respect for the life he had lived, the love he had known, and the holy passage he had just made.

The chaplain's work does not end with the final breath. We hold space for those who remain, tending to the immediate waves of grief. We ensure the practical steps are taken with dignity. We embody calm and care until the family is ready for the next part of their journey.

Holding space for someone's departure is one of the most sacred privileges in spiritual care. It changes you. It humbles you. It teaches you, again and again, that death is not simply an ending, but a threshold.

And you carry these moments with you, not as a weight, but as a sacred trust.

CHAPTER 10

AFTER DEATH — BLESSING, COMMITTAL, AND CONTINUING CARE

Death does not signal the conclusion of the chaplain's work. It does not draw a line under the story. Rather, it ushers in a new chapter, one that centres on the living. In the hours and days after a patient's passing, the chaplain remains a steady, compassionate presence for those who grieve: the family, the friends, and even the members of staff whose own hearts are touched by the loss. The ministry continues, still sacred, still gentle, but now directed towards those left behind.

After Kojo's final breath, the atmosphere in the room shifted. The silence was different now. It no longer carried the tense anticipation of waiting; instead, it held the soft, unalterable weight of finality. Ama sat beside her father's bed, her hand resting over his, tracing the familiar lines of fingers she had once held as a child. Her tears had slowed, yet she clung to that touch. She was not ready to leave, and there was no need for her to hurry.

I spoke quietly.

"Would you like us to say a blessing before the body is taken?"

She nodded, her voice barely audible.

"Please."

Standing at Kojo's bedside, I placed my hand gently on his shoulder and prayed:

"Holy God, we thank You for the life of Kojo, for every memory treasured, every moment shared, every expression of love given and received. Receive him now into Your eternal care. May his soul be at peace, and may those who love him find comfort and strength in You. Amen."

Ama whispered, "Thank you."

Blessings after death are never for the departed alone. They are also for the living, for the ones who must now carry the weight of absence. These words help to frame the unspoken, to acknowledge the sacredness of the moment, and to affirm the hope that death is not the end. For some, it is a prayer of release; for others, a benediction over a love that will never truly fade.

After the blessing, I stepped quietly from the room to give Ama and the family space to sit with their grief. Later, I returned to offer further support, whether that meant guidance in funeral planning, ongoing pastoral visits, or simply a listening ear in the days to come.

Chaplains are often invited to take part in committal services. These may take place at a hospital bedside, in the quiet of a family home, or at the graveside. They are brief, yet profound moments of closure. They honour the body, mark the transition from life to death, and help those present take the first step in the long and uneven journey of mourning.

In Kojo's case, Ama later told me he had made a request before his death: that I speak at his funeral.

"He trusted you," she said. "He found peace because you walked with him."

It was one of the deepest honours of my ministry.

But the chaplain's role after death reaches further still, to the healthcare staff. Doctors, nurses, care assistants, porters, cleaners, all can form quiet bonds with patients they have served for days, weeks, or even months. Their grief is often unacknowledged, tucked away in order to carry on with the next patient, the next shift.

Shortly after Kojo's passing, I went to the nurses' station. One of them looked up and said with a sad smile:

"He was a good man. Stubborn, yes, but kind. I'll miss him."

We spoke for a while, sharing memories, allowing space for emotion. In those moments, we were not processing a case; we were remembering a person. This is a kind of debriefing, not born of protocol, but of shared humanity.

Grief is not the sole property of the immediate family. It touches every soul who has walked part of the journey with the dying.

Part of the chaplain's vocation is to recognise this, to bless it, and to allow it room to breathe.

Sometimes this ongoing care takes the form of a follow-up call or letter. Sometimes it means attending a memorial service. And sometimes, it is simply the quiet reassurance of, "I remember too."

The work of chaplaincy after death is delicate. It is deeply relational. It offers no quick fixes, no forced optimism. It provides presence, a safe space in which grief is honoured, memories are sacred, and hope is offered, however gently.

Kojo's death left a space in the lives of those who loved him. But it did not leave a void. In that space remain love, memory, and the grace of reconciliation, seeds that will continue to bear fruit in the lives of those who remain. As his chaplain, I was privileged not only to witness his journey, but to honour it beyond his final breath.

This is the unending rhythm of the work: one life, one death, one story at a time. And each story, like each soul, is sacred.

CHAPTER 11

THE CHAPLAIN'S OWN GRIEF AND GROWTH

Healthcare chaplains are trained to hold space for others, to stand beside families in distress, to accompany the dying, and to remain steady in the midst of emotional storms. Yet what is less often spoken of is the quiet, private grief that chaplains themselves carry. For in walking alongside others through the valley of death, we are not untouched. We are changed. We are marked, sometimes in ways that stay with us for life.

Kojo's death lingered in my thoughts and heart long after the room was cleared, after the chart was signed off, and after the hospital corridors returned to their usual hum. I would remember his voice, sometimes weary, sometimes curious, sometimes brave. I would recall his questions, the way his eyes softened in those final days, the hesitant but tender reunion with Ama. I remembered the Psalm he had asked me to read, and how my own voice trembled as I spoke the words at his bedside.

Chaplains are not immune to grief. We do not simply pass from one room to the next, unmarked by what we witness. We carry fragments of every story, sometimes quietly in our minds, often deeply in our hearts. And though each encounter leaves its imprint, some, like Kojo's, become part of who we are.

There is a grief particular to this work. It is not the sharp, devastating loss of a close relative or dear friend; it is quieter, more layered, often mixed with gratitude. It is the grief of seeing humanity in its most vulnerable form. The grief of saying goodbye over and over again. The grief of walking with someone to the very threshold of life, only to step back as they cross alone.

And yet, alongside the grief, there is growth.

Each end-of-life journey reshapes the chaplain. It refines our understanding of presence. It stretches our capacity for compassion. It humbles us. We are confronted, again and again, with life's fragility, and with it, a sharper sense of what truly matters: love offered and received, forgiveness extended, dignity preserved, peace embraced.

For me, the grief I carry as a chaplain is not a weight to be resented, but a sacred inheritance. It reminds me that I was entrusted with someone's last days. That I was allowed into moments where masks fell away and truth was spoken without pretence. That I stood in rooms where eternity brushed against time, and I bore witness to it.

But such closeness requires care. Self-care is not a luxury in this work; it is a necessity. Without it, grief becomes cumulative, and the well of compassion can run dry.

For me, grieving well means making time for reflection and prayer. It means engaging in spiritual direction and seeking honest conversations with trusted colleagues who understand the unique weight of this calling. It means rest, the kind of rest that is intentional, restorative, and not apologised for. It means letting the sadness do its work of shaping me, without allowing it to hollow me out.

I have my own small rituals for the patients who have died. Sometimes I light a candle in their memory. Sometimes I write their name in a private journal reserved for such remembrances. Sometimes I read a Psalm they loved, or simply sit in stillness, letting the memory of them fill the silence. These acts do not erase the grief; they sanctify it. They remind me that I am not simply a professional providing a service, but a human being who has been given the privilege of walking on holy ground.

And on that holy ground, growth happens.

Kojo taught me lessons no training manual could convey. He reminded me that even those who feel far from God are never beyond God's reach. That reconciliation, however improbable, can come in life's final chapter. That steady, patient presence can accomplish what medicine alone cannot.

His story has become part of my story.

This, I think, is one of the profound mysteries of chaplaincy: we walk with others so that they may find peace, and in doing so, we ourselves are transformed. Our hearts widen. Our faith deepens. Our ability to love, and to grieve, becomes richer.

This work is not easy. It costs something. But it is holy. And if I were asked again to choose this path, knowing both the grief and the grace it brings, I would say yes, every time.

CHAPTER 12

REFLECTIONS ON PRACTICE — THEOLOGICAL AND PRACTICAL INSIGHTS

The journey with Kojo was more than a pastoral encounter; it was a profound meeting of humanity, faith, and grace. His story, a tapestry of presence, reconciliation, and a quiet rediscovery of faith, became a lens through which to reflect on the wider truths of chaplaincy and end-of-life care.

This chapter steps back from the personal narrative to explore both the theological foundations and the practical realities of what it means to serve as a chaplain in that sacred threshold where life meets death.

1. Death Is Not Merely Medical — It Is Spiritual

Modern healthcare systems are often shaped around clinical observation and intervention. The focus, understandably, is on physical decline, monitoring vital signs, adjusting treatment, relieving pain. Yet death is never simply a biological process; it is also a profoundly human and spiritual moment.

It is the culmination of a lifetime's relationships, choices, memories, and hopes. It carries mystery and meaning far beyond the reach of medical instruments.

For the chaplain, recognising this is central. We are not there to treat symptoms, but to care for souls. When the work of medicine has reached its limit, the work of the spirit begins in earnest, tending to dignity, offering love, and helping a person let go in peace.

2. Theology Must Be Lived, Not Only Taught

Chaplains draw deeply on theology: the nature of God, the promise of eternity, the purpose of suffering, the hope of redemption. But in the intimate space of the bedside, theology must be more than doctrine, it must be embodied.

With Kojo, there were no sermons. Instead, I sought to live the truths I believe: God's nearness, His compassion, His unrelenting presence. Theology in that moment was not a lecture; it was a quiet reading of a Psalm, a hand held without hurry, a prayer spoken in trust.

The most powerful theological statement I could make was not, "Here is the explanation," but, "God is here. Even now. Even here."

3. Presence Is Powerful

One of the defining lessons of chaplaincy is that people do not always need, or even want, eloquent words. They need presence. Steady, compassionate, non-anxious presence.

It is presence that gives people courage to voice their fears. Presence that holds the space for forgiveness to be sought and offered. Presence that bears witness when life's end draws near and the room becomes charged with meaning.

In a world filled with constant noise, the chaplain's presence offers a countercultural gift: the stillness to be fully there for another human being.

4. Spiritual Pain Is Real — And Must Be Addressed

Kojo's deepest suffering was not his diagnosis. It was the regret, the unresolved relationships, the yearning to be at peace with his story. These were not simply psychological matters; they were spiritual wounds.

Recognising spiritual pain requires attentive listening and discernment. Addressing it requires patience, gentleness, and the refusal to rush the process. When spiritual wounds are acknowledged and tended to, physical pain often becomes more bearable, because the whole person is being honoured.

5. Interdisciplinary Collaboration Is Essential

End-of-life care is never a solo effort. Doctors, nurses, social workers, and chaplains all bring unique perspectives.

The chaplain's role in this team is to ensure that the spiritual and emotional needs of the patient are not overlooked. This requires both humility and courage, the humility to recognise the expertise of others, and the courage to speak when the voice of the soul risks being drowned out by the busyness of clinical care.

When the interdisciplinary team values the chaplain's contribution, care becomes holistic, addressing body, mind, and spirit together.

6. Self-Care Is Sacred Stewardship

As reflected in the previous chapter, the emotional and spiritual weight of this work is immense. Without healthy rhythms of reflection, prayer, and rest, chaplains risk burnout or compassion fatigue.

Self-care is not self-indulgence; it is stewardship. It is the tending of one's own soul so that we can continue to tend the souls of others. This may involve spiritual direction, retreats, honest conversations with peers, or simply allowing ourselves to rest without guilt.

7. Every Patient Is a Teacher

Over the years, I have learnt to approach every patient, regardless of background or beliefs, as a teacher.

Kojo taught me the power of reconciliation in the final chapter of life. Others have taught me the courage to face death without fear, the strength of faith under pressure, or the beauty of joy in the midst of pain.

The chaplain is never only a giver of care. We are also lifelong students of the sacred, learning with every encounter, and growing with every goodbye.

Chaplaincy at the end of life is not an optional extra. It is a vital, sacred ministry that brings humanity, hope, and a sense of the holy into one of life's most vulnerable passages. It affirms that every person matters, right up to their final breath.

And for those of us who serve in this role, it offers a paradoxical gift: in caring for the dying, we are invited closer to the mystery of life itself, to its fragility, its beauty, and its eternal significance.

CONCLUSION

DEATH AS HOLY GROUND

Death is not merely an ending; it is a threshold, a veil, a sacred passage. For those of us called to serve as chaplains, it is a place where we instinctively remove our shoes, for the ground beneath our feet is holy.

Walking with Kojo through the final stretch of his earthly life was not simply a professional responsibility. It was a profound privilege, a sacred honour. He entrusted me with his fears, his memories, his hopes, and his grief. He allowed me to bear witness not only to his dying, but also to his becoming. And in doing so, he left an indelible mark upon my soul.

Every dying patient is a mirror, reflecting something of the shared human condition. They remind us that we are far more than our diagnoses, accomplishments, or possessions. At the edge of life, what endures is love, love given, love received, love remembered.

The work of a healthcare chaplain is often quiet, almost invisible, yet deeply significant. We walk hospital corridors and sit in palliative care rooms, not with ready-made answers, but with presence. We offer no cures, yet we offer comfort. We do not remove the sting of death, yet we stand within it, so that others do not have to stand there alone.

In the course of writing this book, and in the countless moments that shaped it, I have become more convinced than ever that death is not our ultimate enemy. It is an integral part of life. It can be approached with dignity, grace, and even beauty.

Yes, death is painful. Yes, it brings sorrow. But it can also bring reconciliation, healing, and unexpected joy. I have seen faith rekindled in a final breath. I have heard forgiveness whispered in hushed, trembling tones. I have witnessed families rediscover one another. And I have sensed the presence of God more acutely in the stillness of death than in the most exuberant sanctuary.

The journey with an end-of-life patient is never about us, yet it changes us. It shapes our spirit, chisels our values, and teaches us to listen without haste, to honour without condition, to hope without fear, and to let go with grace.

Kojo reminded me, as so many patients have, that every life is a story worth telling, every death is a doorway worth respecting, and every moment in between is a gift worth receiving.

So, let us walk slowly. Let us speak gently. Let us listen deeply. Let us stand in the sacred silence of the dying and recognise, with unshakable certainty, that we are on holy ground.

And let us never forget: Even in death, there is light. Even in grief, there is grace. Even in silence, God speaks.

APPENDICES

APPENDIX A: SAMPLE PRAYERS AND BLESSINGS

1. Prayer for Peace at the End of Life. God of mercy and grace, As this life draws to a close, surround Your beloved child with peace. Still the mind, calm the heart, and fill this room with Your gentle presence. May fear dissolve into trust, and may there be no striving, only rest in You. Amen.

2. Prayer for the Dying. Holy One, as the veil thins and eternity draws near, Be present with this soul who has walked the path of life with courage and dignity. Hold them now in Your everlasting arms. Let the light of Your love guide them home. Amen.

3. Final Blessing After Death. Into Your hands, O Lord, we commend this precious soul. May they rest from their labours and rise in glory. Surround those who mourn with comfort, and sustain them with hope. Let peace reign in this place of parting, and may love endure beyond the grave. Amen.

APPENDIX

B: INTERFAITH CONSIDERATIONS IN END-OF-LIFE CHAPLAINCY

Healthcare chaplains often work within pluralistic environments, serving individuals and families from a wide range of spiritual, religious, and cultural backgrounds. In such contexts, respectful and inclusive care is essential.

> ➢ **Key Principles for Interfaith Chaplaincy:**

- **Ask, don't assume.** Approach with gentle curiosity: "Can you tell me

about your spiritual or cultural preferences at this time?"
- **Begin with neutral language.** For example: "Would you like someone to sit with you?" rather than "Shall I pray for you?"
- **Collaborate with other faith leaders.** If a patient requests a ritual or rite you are not trained to lead, facilitate contact with their own spiritual representative.
- **Be mindful of cultural sensitivities.** Respect traditions relating to touch, gender roles, modesty, death rituals, and post-mortem care.
- **Offer spiritual care without proselytising.** Chaplaincy is about accompaniment and support, not persuasion or conversion.

➢ **Interfaith End-of-Life Phrases:**

- "Would you like me to sit quietly with you?"

- "Is there a prayer, reading, or tradition that would bring you comfort?"
- "Would you like me to help you contact your religious leader or community?"

Creating an atmosphere of safety and respect makes the chaplain become a bridge between the medical setting and the sacred traditions that bring meaning to the patient and their loved ones.

APPENDIX C: SELF-CARE RESOURCES FOR CHAPLAINS

Chaplains carry sacred burdens. Without intentional care, the weight can lead to compassion fatigue, burnout, or emotional numbness. Attending to one's own spiritual and emotional wellbeing is not indulgence, it is stewardship of the calling.

➢ **Signs You May Need to Pause:**

- Emotional detachment or numbness
- Loss of empathy, irritability, or cynicism
- Difficulty sleeping or concentrating
- Diminished joy or fulfilment in ministry
- Feeling persistently exhausted or overwhelmed

➢ **Self-Care Practices:**

1. **Regular Spiritual Direction or Supervision** – Engage with someone skilled in listening to and guiding your spiritual journey.
2. **Peer Debriefing** – Set aside intentional time with colleagues to process intense encounters and share mutual support.
3. **Sabbath Rest** – Dedicate time that is neither pastoral nor clinical; allow it to be truly restorative.

4. **Creative Expression** – Write, paint, garden, sing, or walk, activities that allow the heart to express what cannot be spoken.
5. **Healthy Boundaries** – Learn the discipline of saying "no" when necessary, and allow yourself to step back for renewal.

A Chaplain's Daily Grounding Prayer: Loving God, today I walk into places of suffering. Keep me from rushing to fix; instead, teach me to pause and truly be present. Let me carry Your light, not by shining my own glory, but by reflecting Yours. Show me how to release what I cannot hold, and to rest when I am weary. Amen.

www.ingramcontent.com/pod-product-compliance
Lightning Source LLC
Chambersburg PA
CBHW060045230426
43661CB00004B/664